The Connection Between Operations and Marketing

Case Studies of the Best Dental Practices

By Ryan Gross

Foreword by Dr. Addison Killeen

2023 Paperback Second Edition

© 2023 Ryan Gross

All rights reserved.

Published in the United States by KDP, an imprint of Amazon.

Library of Congress Cataloging-in-Publication Data

Gross, Ryan.

Operations and Marketing: How They Work Together To Create The Dental Practice of Your Dreams / by Ryan Gross

ISBN: 9798394830501

1. Dentistry 2. Dental Office Practice

ABOUT THE AUTHOR

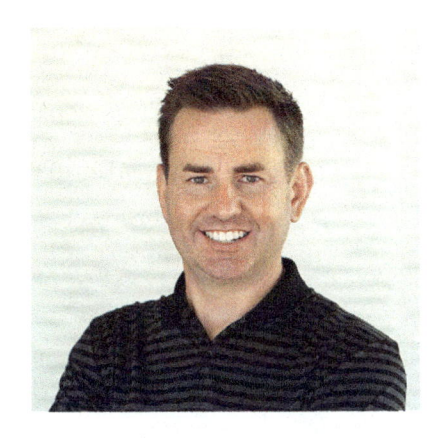

Ryan is the marketing expert and CEO of CMOShare. He has 15+ years of marketing, brand management, communications, and sales experience working with The Walt Disney Company and other large visitor attractions.

After leaving the attraction industry, he consulted with the dental and medical industry to increase patient satisfaction. In 2019, he founded CMOShare to focus specifically on empowering dental practices and small business owners. His proven techniques have increased revenue through marketing and communication strategies. He has managed multiple million-dollar budgets and helped dental practices increase new patient acquisition and patient retention.

TABLE OF CONTENTS

Foreword

Introduction

Chapter 1: Keith + Associates

Chapter 2: Mount Vernon Smile Design

Chapter 3: Broad Smiles Pediatric and Orthodontics

Chapter 4: Humlicek Family Dental

Chapter 5: Finger Lakes Dental Care

Chapter 6: MFD Dental

Chapter 7: Summit Family Dentistry

Chapter 8: Moorehead Family Dentistry

Chapter 9: What Makes a Great Practice?

FORWARD

In early 2019, as I was driving past my favorite sandwich shop, I noticed it was closed and empty. Although I was disappointed about missing out on their 'Thanksgiving Dinner' sandwich, which was made with turkey, dressing, and gravy, I was more so excited about the idea of leasing the space for a dental start-up. I called up the realtor and stated my case and desire to lease the space. A few weeks later, I signed the purchase contracts and began construction on my new dental office.

When I finally started my dental practice in the fall of 2019, I was optimistic about the outcomes of my newfound freedom in my own little shop. As things got underway, I leaned on my friends in town to help me design everything in the practice, particularly Ryan Gross. Ryan and I have been friends for years, and he helped me match the internal decor to my logo, as well as the overall feel of the practice. Although Ryan was still fully employed as the Chief Marketing Officer of a local zoo, I bought him beers and coffee as a token of appreciation for his assistance throughout the process. He constantly reminded me of the importance of setting the right brand, telling a good story, and making sure all pieces of the marketing puzzle worked together. There were many times when he steered me clear of some crazy idea I had, and it paid off big time.

Initially, I used a large national company to create my website. I planned to spend quite a bit of money on marketing my new practice so I could gain quick traction on visibility in a saturated market. I invested in billboards, mailers, and lots of internal marketing. The billboards were a hit, and the mailers got my name out there. Although the website looked aesthetically pleasing, it took me months to realize that there were problems lurking below the surface.

As a start-up, I was willing to put in the hard work to gain new patients. However, I began sensing something was off when a Sunday morning emergency patient asked for the location of my office. I left church early, went to the practice to help this young gal, and was patiently waiting for her to arrive. She called a second time, asking, "Where is your practice again?" I told her the cross-streets again- which are pretty easy to remember since it's 2 of the most major streets in Lincoln, Nebraska. After confirming her location, it turned out she lived in California, and was looking for a dentist in Los Angeles! I thought it was just weird, but maybe a fluke?

A few weeks later, while on Facebook, I noticed that Facebook had generated a possible advertisement that they thought I should use. However, it said "Dentist in San Bernardino," which looked odd enough that I had to do some digging to find out why Facebook thought that my practice was in San Bernardino, California. After enlisting Ryan's help, I found out that my website was an exact copy of another dentist-client of this website company, located in California. Although the pictures and some of the text were mine, the metadata and other "invisible" information were all based around a different doctor in a different city. Even though I thought this was a custom site for me, it was actually telling the digital universe that I was 1,500 miles away.

However, when I looked at my data, I thought the site must have still been performing well because I could see the traffic. After discussing with Ryan, he showed me that the data portal this company created hides a lot of details, such as where the traffic is coming from. It turns out that I was a HUGE hit in California.

When I called this company to discuss the issues, they had no answer. This left me frustrated and depressed, that I had spent close to $100,000 on marketing for my startup and my website had not been optimized for my city.

After a few tumultuous months, I asked Ryan to build me my own custom website, with access to my own data. Fortunately, he agreed, and I am now able to sleep better knowing that I can see the actual data and that my site is performing well. Soon after helping me, he started helping other dentists and creating his own company.

Even beyond seeing my data for myself, I've always been impressed by the fact that CMOshare is willing to dive deep into the numbers to determine whether marketing is even warranted and is there an actual return to gain from a marketing investment. They are truly my outsourced Chief Marketing Officer and even though I give the guidance, they are the ones who determine who and when marketing will work for my practice.

Dr. Addison Killeen
Co-Founder of Dental Success Network
Author of 'By The Numbers' and
The Dental Success Manuals
Host of the Daily Dental Podcast

INTRODUCTION

This book is not intended to dive into the intricacies of marketing, reveal the insider secrets of how some dentists have transformed their fledgling practices into multi-million-dollar enterprises, or highlight the most innovative marketing strategies. Nor is it intended to help you attract 200 new patients each month. If that is what you are looking for, then this is not the book for you. You may as well leave it on your shelf to gather dust.

The primary objective of this book is to focus on how marketing connects to operations. Not the mundane, run-of-the-mill operations, but the most captivating systems and processes that are being used in dental clinics all over the country. The dentists we have interviewed for this book are highly skilled operators, the Navy SEALS of the dental world. They are problem-solvers who possess laser-like precision, coupled with a panoramic view of the dental landscape. They are adept at spotting opportunities from afar and then leveraging marketing strategies to achieve their goals.

These dentists understand when and how to market, as well as when not to. While they may be frugal in their pursuit of success, they also know when it is necessary to spend money freely in order to test new ideas. While many of their innovative ideas may not have worked out, they double down on the ones that do, ultimately achieving gains that far outweigh their past failures.

The dentists featured in this book are among the best in the business. By generously sharing their data, we can demonstrate how operations and marketing are inextricably linked. Without effective operations, marketing efforts can be wasteful, akin to a drunken gambler in a casino, spending money without any clear way to track its impact. Marketing that overloads an underdeveloped system with too many patients can quickly lead to disaster. Likewise, marketing that only allows a small stream of water to break out of the faucet can dry up funds and time without ever providing any value. Neither case is ideal.

Conversely, operations without marketing are like a Ferrari with an empty fuel tank. It may look beautiful, but it is useless if you can't drive it anywhere. Similarly, a great dental practice with no patients is not a great practice at all. We aim to strike a balance between the two, to demonstrate the connections between operations and marketing, and to glean insights from top performers in the field. We hope you enjoy this book.

KEY TAKEAWAYS

In the following case studies, you will find differences and similarities. Some factors hold true across each strategy and others are invariably different due to unique factors such as practice location, competition, market conditions and operational needs. To make it really easy to understand what's what, we've included a brief overview of each component that is part of the success of each case study.

Market Share

You will notice that market share is mentioned often throughout these case studies. Our goal is to create the highest online market share possible for each practice that we work with. To do this we want to rank in search results, primarily on Google, for long-tail key phrases (often called key terms) that have the highest value for the practice and quickest impact on growth.

We also define value as a quality patient conversion. This is an important definition to unfold–value is not in *any* conversion, it's in *quality* conversions–something many marketing companies don't distinguish between.

The next question, naturally is, so, what keywords have the most value? Typically, a higher value search term is related to a higher value sale, or more profitable service. So, for example, converting organically for "wisdom teeth removal" is worth more because it has a higher production value to your practice.

The "most valuable market share" for each practice has some elements that are the same across the foundation, and others that may vary depending on objective, practice location, etc. For example, a practice in California is going to have a possible market share that is vastly different from a practice in Nebraska simply because California has a much higher saturation rate of dentists than Nebraska. This may mean that the market share for certain specialty services should be the focus for a practice in Los Angeles, where market share for new hygiene patients should be the focus for a practice in Nebraska.

Another common misconception is the desire or need to rank number one in searches such as "dentist near me" or "dentist in "city name here." Those searches are highly valuable to rank in on page one as they may make up 30% or so of the market searches. But we must remember that there are still **70% of searches available** and within that 70%, there is an opportunity to steal the market in "wisdom teeth removal," or "emergency dental," or "dental implants," or many other smaller search terms that no one else cares about. This means you could focus on key search terms that are more profitable and sometimes easier to capture.

It's also important to mention that search engines are continuously changing the algorithm around local searches. Where it used to matter to enter "dentist near me," now, Google is smart enough to know where the user is and serve up the practice in closest proximity first, without a "near me" search. This is something you have no control over, but greatly affects how often your site will come up to the top of the list. Now if users are searching with "near me" in the keyphrase we want to optimize for it, but we also want to ensure our reliance upon it diminishes at the same rate that Google's reliance upon it diminishes.

Web traffic = Phone Calls = New Patients/Production

We've tracked marketing and operational data for over 100 dental practices in North America for the past two years. Ninety-four of the practices showed a correlation between web traffic, phone calls, and new patient/production. This is a lead KPI and should be used as the foundation of monitoring your marketing success.

This follows a train-of-thought pattern that is typical for marketing in almost every area of society, from museums to restaurants to dental offices. A potential client needs a product, your business comes to the top of their mind, they search for your business, check out your website or Facebook page, and then they finally call your office.

If your office answers the phone, has a great experience on the phone, and is also able to satisfy the needs of that client, then this patient might have a good chance of choosing your business. This sounds simple, but it is actually a difficult situation to have enough staffing that can answer most phone calls. Then you have to train up the staff to be prepared for each type of phone call, with enough knowledge to answer all the needs of the caller. After you answer their call and address their needs, then they might be interested enough in you to want to schedule.

However, this leads to the final operational hiccup that can occur- Can you schedule these new patients in a timely manner? The best dental practices we see often use Block Scheduling to allow for patient blocks to make scheduling easier. This means saving blocks of time for new patients and emergencies, but some high-performing dentists even do blockouts for crown seats, simple fillings, multiple fillings, crowns, and implants. The more detailed your block scheduling, the more you can plan your day around the flow that works for you.

Operational Needs

Ensuring your marketing and operations are working together is critical to your overall success. A high answer rate of inbound calls, optimized scheduling, and knowing what type of patient you are looking for is imperative to getting it right. For instance, if you have limited capacity, you don't want to focus on new general patients, instead you want to focus on dental emergencies and higher value services that will allow you to optimize production. Conversely, if you have hygiene availability for new patients but focus on specialty services, you are not increasing your active patient base and possible long-term production–making it harder to achieve stable, long-term growth.

When we think of operations, we think not only of getting more patients in your door, but also what you do with them once they are in your chair. The best dentists make sure that the educated patient is already primed to get their dental needs fixed. If they need an implant, we want to already pre-sell that your dental practice is the perfect place that can help them. If they need financing, the best operational dentists are already prepared with options to create easy monthly payment plans.

CHAPTER 1

Keith + Associates Dentistry

Location - Mission, Kansas (Kansas City Area)
Doctors - 6
Annual Production - $8 million

Practice Overview

Keith + Associates Dentistry is a general practice located in Mission, Kansas, with a focus on sedation, implants, and surgery. The practice is owned by Dr. Bill Keith and his wife Ashley and is built upon a foundation of providing an informative and comforting patient experience. The practice has a large and very active patient base and has recently opened a surgical center that focuses on full-mouth implants and surgery.

Challenge and Growth Opportunity

Keith + Associates Dentistry is a large, very successful practice that was looking to continue growing its patient base through hygiene while also expanding beyond general dentistry. Managing this strategy was critical to the future growth of the practice. In this case study, we detail the correlation between website traffic, website conversions, phone calls, and new patients.

The most successful practices we work with have a huge focus on increasing their active patient base. This journey usually begins with increasing hygiene patients. Then, once new hygiene patients are maxed or close to maxed out due to office capacity, population of the area, competition, operation of the practice, etc. the next step for increasing revenue is growing market share around higher value treatments. In Keith + Associates' case, the practice was underperforming from a marketing standpoint, had a lower phone answer rate, and needed to establish the surgery and sedation brand of the practice.

The Work

When we first started working with the Keith's, the goal was to optimize new patients through hygiene, increase implant cases, and promote sedation dentistry services at the practice. We started with the bread and butter–focusing on hygiene and expanding the active patient base. To do this we needed to increase local web visits and conversions. Secondarily, we needed to begin work on both an implant and sedation marketing strategy that would drive awareness and conversions through these two specialty services.

To start, we built a new website with a focus on gaining an increase in local web traffic and phone conversions. We know from past experience that in most cases, when we can increase local web visitors we can increase conversions, which equates to more phone calls, which equals new patients, and thereby leads to increased production. The term "local" is extremely important here. If website traffic is increased but that traffic is outside the geographic area, i.e., not local, then traffic does not equal phone calls. Why would someone in California care about a search result of a dentist in Nebraska? Demographics of search results is a common area that gets missed–and that miss has a huge impact on results.

The Results

Once the new website, Google and social ads were launched we started tracking marketing and operations metrics. After two months we noticed local web traffic and online conversion increasing, which is fantastic, but new patient numbers were not keeping up at the same pace. So, we had a disconnect somewhere.

We began looking deeper into the numbers and found inbound phone calls (by number) were increasing, but the answer rate of those calls was low. Essentially, the phone was ringing, but the calls were not being answered.

To re-verify our calculations on outcomes in response to actions, we laid out the following truths:

- The Keith's had a new patient goal of 135 to 145 a month.
- Efforts had increased phone conversions from the website by 30%
- The practice was receiving a total number of 2,200 calls per month.
- Average answer rate is 85% and average conversion rate is 8%.

Based upon an answer rate of 85%, 2,200 calls would equal 150 new patients. However, a shortage of employees at the front desk was creating a call answer percentage lower than 85%.

This proved that if we could get their web visits to 2,200 per month, and they were able to hire 1-2 more front desk employees, then we would most likely see their new patients above 145 patients per month.

This brought up an important point - too many offices focus on generating marketing, but don't have enough team members to answer the phones. Once Keith + Associates realized they had a problem, they quickly added team members to answer the phones.

As expected, web traffic and conversions increased, as well as inbound phone call answer percentage. The attached graph shows the correlation between web traffic, inbound calls, new patients and production. You will see a near identical increase in inbound phone calls and new patients and production. Note that the larger increase in web traffic increases at a higher rate. This is due to All-on-X implant marketing that included a heavy social media ad strategy.

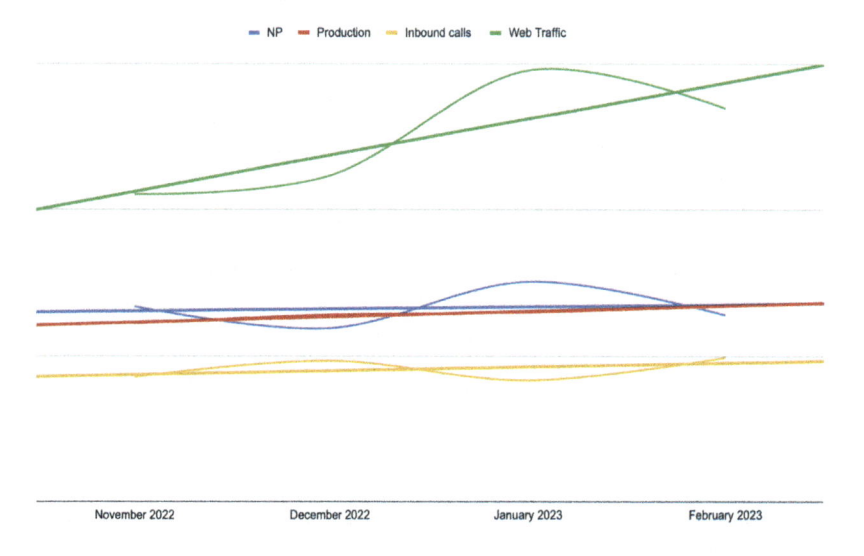

The increase in new patients occurred quickly once web traffic and inbound calls increased, which happened relatively quickly.

Once the practice was starting to fill with more regular new patients, then we could focus on specialty dentistry. The second part of the strategy was to increase overall production through All-on-X implant marketing and sedation. The All-on-X marketing plan has a longer implementation period and conversion process. However, to increase production quicker, we've also started to increase awareness for sedation dentistry.

Full Mouth Dental Implants

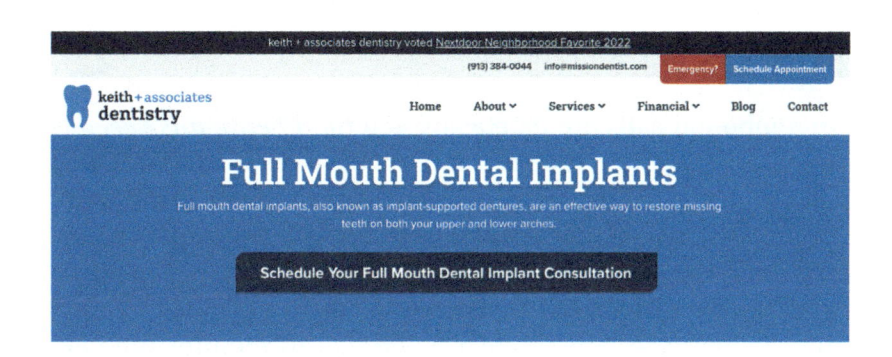

Full mouth dental implants, also known as implant-supported dentures, are an effective way to restore missing teeth on both your upper and lower arches.

Schedule Your Full Mouth Dental Implant Consultation

Full Mouth Dental Implants from Keith + Associates

Full-mouth dental implants are an alternative to dentures. This method requires only four implants per jaw, compared to traditional implants that require eight to ten implants per jaw. The full-mouth dental implant technique reduces the need for bone grafting and the implants act just like natural teeth, making this procedure quicker, easier, and more comfortable for patients. keith + associates dentistry is proud to offer expert-level full-mouth dental implants to Mission, KS, and the surrounding communities.

Visit Our Implant Center Site

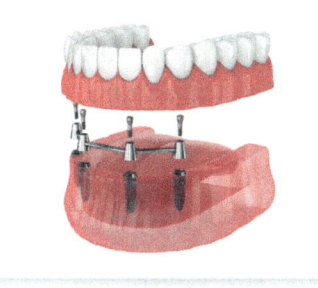

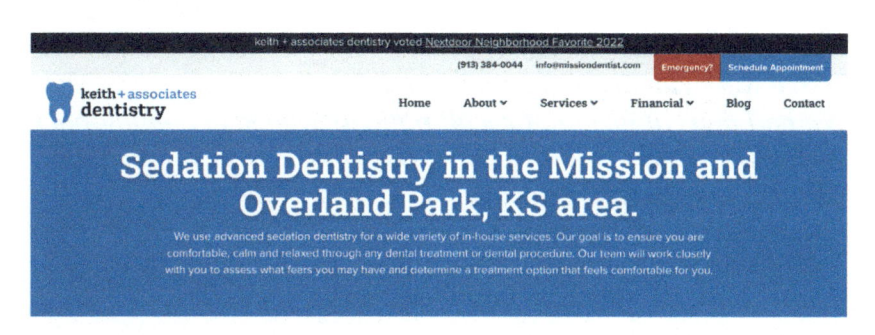

Sedation Dentistry in the Mission and Overland Park, KS area.

We use advanced sedation dentistry for a wide variety of in-house services. Our goal is to ensure you are comfortable, calm and relaxed through any dental treatment or dental procedure. Our team will work closely with you to assess what fears you may have and determine a treatment option that feels comfortable for you.

The Purpose of Dental Sedation

Sedation dentistry is the use of any type of dental sedation to reduce stress, anxiety, and any physical pain associated with dental treatment. Sedation is a safe and convenient way to help you feel more relaxed while at the dentist's while your treatment is being completed. We offer dental sedation through laughing gas, oral conscious, and IV sedation. IV sedation is most commonly used at keith + associates dentistry for surgical procedures, such as wisdom teeth removal or dental implants.

It's important that you feel comfortable and safe during your procedure. Before any procedure, your doctor will recommend the appropriate level of sedation that meets your needs. Then, we will set up your appointment and plan accordingly for your procedure, knowing that you will be relaxed and calm during the dental appointment.

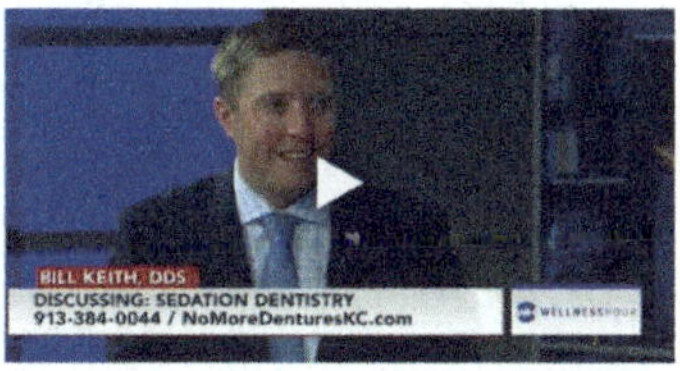

Schedule an Appointment Online

Conclusion

Ensuring inbound calls are increasing and ***then being answered*** is critical to growing new patient and active patient numbers and production. These data points correlate directly with each other and ensure that marketing conversions are equaling actual new patients. Increasing web traffic is the first step in this process followed by conversions on the website. Once this occurs, inbound calls will increase. At this point it is critical to monitor inbound phone call answer rates. Increasing web traffic and inbound phone calls should be an immediate priority, followed by a long-term strategy for higher production through implant, sedation and other high value service marketing.

From Dr. Bill Keith

'When I initially purchased my practice the marketing budget was zero. We were running at capacity and didn't really see a need for it. We had a great group of recall patients who kept coming back religiously for their re-care, but rarely had significant treatment needed. As we started growing the footprint of the practice, we began to start marketing. What we found is that by marketing, we drastically increase the production numbers for our doctors because these new patients had a significant amount of treatment that was needed.

When we began working with Ryan and his team, we were introduced to marketing data. Prior it had been a shotgun and shoot from the hip approach. It was working, but it was inefficient and got us a lot of prospects that were strong. Such as patients who were seeking middle of the night emergency treatment which we do not provide. Once we began working with true market data, we were able to target our ideal audience and attract the patients we wanted while largely eliminating those which were not our ideal candidates.

We began offering more and more new patient appointments because we could see that there was a direct correlation between the number of new patients we got and the productivity of our doctors. It's been really fun to watch and tweak the different aspects of this as we continue to grow the practice.

Key Takeaways:

- Increasing Web presence brings increasing phone calls
- Ensuring you have staff to answer phone calls is critical
- Tracking local vs non-local web visits ensures your marketing to the right market
- Capacity of the practice will change your marketing focus from hygiene new patients to emergencies, implants, and more exotic types of dental services.

CHAPTER 2

Mount Vernon Smile Design

Location - Mount Vernon, Washington
Doctors - 2
Annual Production - $1.5 million

Practice Overview

Mount Vernon Smile Design is a general practice in Mount Vernon, Washington that focuses on bread-and-butter dentistry. Owned by Dr. Nicholas Forsythe and Dr. Whitney Forsythe, the practice is working on expanding the patient base and including more specialized services such as implants and clear aligners. The Forsythe's have focused the unique value proposition of the practice on being locally owned and having strong ties to the community.

Challenge and Growth Opportunity

Dr. Nicholas Forsythe and Dr. Whitney Forsythe have a unique setup with their dental practice–they are a two-doctor practice with the flexibility of a one doctor owner. They have been able to grow their practice to a $1.5 million dollar business. The practice is built around flexibility and the ability for Dr. Whitney to take time away from the practice as a new mother with Dr. Nicholas filling in for her. We took this business approach and mirrored it in the marketing approach. Our overall goal is to increase hygiene patients, total active patient base and focus on emergencies to increase production per patient. We've done this by working around the needs of the practice depending on the time and situation.

The Work

When we first started working with the practice our goal was to update the branding, establish a greater online presence and create a strong community presence. We created an online strategy to increase market share through organic rankings. The community the practice is located in is an hour north of Seattle and is growing quickly. The competition in the area when we started, in terms of marketing, was low, so we were able to see an increase in online visibility fairly quickly after launching their new website. The site was averaging around 300 web visits a month and after three months increased to nearly 600. This increase was primarily due to a lack of online presence from any other dental practice. Winning at this early stage was easy, but as the complexity increased, so did the competition.

Prior to the website change the practice was averaging around 15 new patients a month. After three months the practice increased new patients to 22 to 25 per month. A focus on emergency services was important to this increase, as their hygiene demand is higher than their capacity. One way to add revenue to the practice in this case is to increase the number of emergency patients on the doctor's schedule.

During this time, we also explored marketing clear aligners externally. After analyzing, we found that conversion rates for clear aligners were much lower than general and emergency conversion rates. After diving into the data and speaking with the practice, we determined that specialty dentistry services in general do not see a high return when marketed externally. Most patients search for a dental office utilizing search and external marketing platforms specifically for general dentistry or emergency dentistry, but not specialty services. In the area, most specialty services were marketed in-house. This led us to focus our online and external marketing strategies exclusively on hygiene and emergencies and focus internally on clear aligners and any other specialty services.

We've also adjusted their brand and logo to reflect the future of the practice. They are in the middle of an expansion that will update the interior to look more modern. With this update, the Forsythe's asked us to update their logo as well. This branding effort will enhance our opportunity to increase marketing efforts internally and externally and ensure we are staying ahead of the competition in the area.

The Original Practice Logo

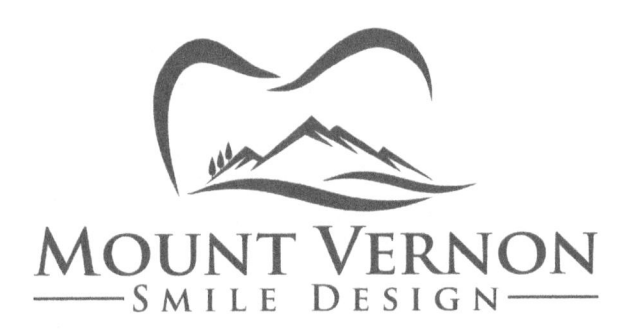

MOUNT VERNON
—— SMILE DESIGN ——

Updated Logo and Website

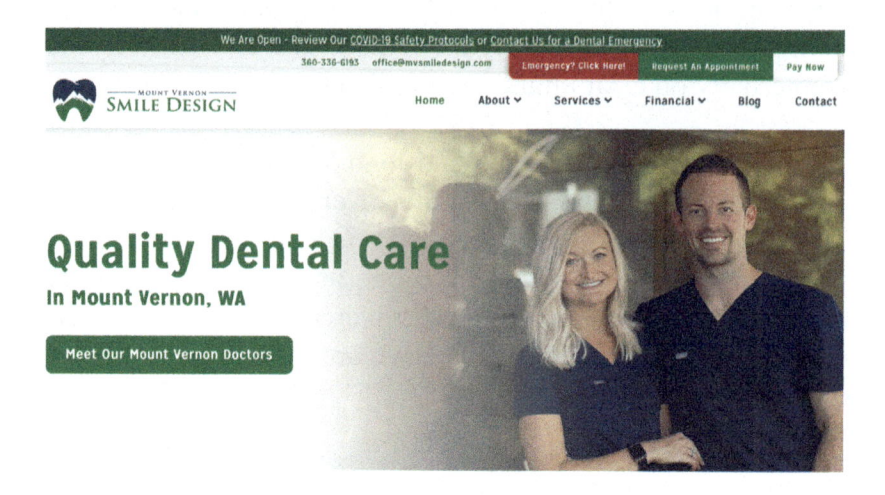

The Result

In the past year, there has been an increase in competition in the area, however, the market share and demand of Mount Vernon Smile Design has consistently increased by the same amount as the competition to keep conversions high. In the past two years, conversions from the website have tripled and kept up with the increase in competition.

One of the key metrics specifically for Mount Vernon Smile Design is the conversion rate. We wanted to measure the number of visitors who took desired actions, such as scheduling an appointment or submitting a "contact us" form. By analyzing web traffic and conversion data, we were able to gain insights into how the practice's website navigation and design affected patient behavior and ultimately impacted the practice's bottom line. We ultimately changed their site layout to increase conversions and focus on the web traffic that was on the site for a longer amount of time.

Looking at the web traffic and conversions graph for Mount Vernon, we noticed a steady increase in web traffic over the course of the year, with a peak in January 2023. This was most likely due to a focused effort on marketing during that time period. While there were fluctuations throughout the year, the overall trend was positive, indicating that our marketing efforts were successful in driving more traffic to the website and converting those visitors into patients.

It's important to note that tracking *online conversions* is just as important as tracking web traffic. By tracking conversions, such as phone calls, appointments scheduled online, and form submissions, we were able to see how many people completed the call-to-actions that the website was designed for. We also took into account where the web traffic was coming from to gauge the effectiveness of our digital marketing efforts.

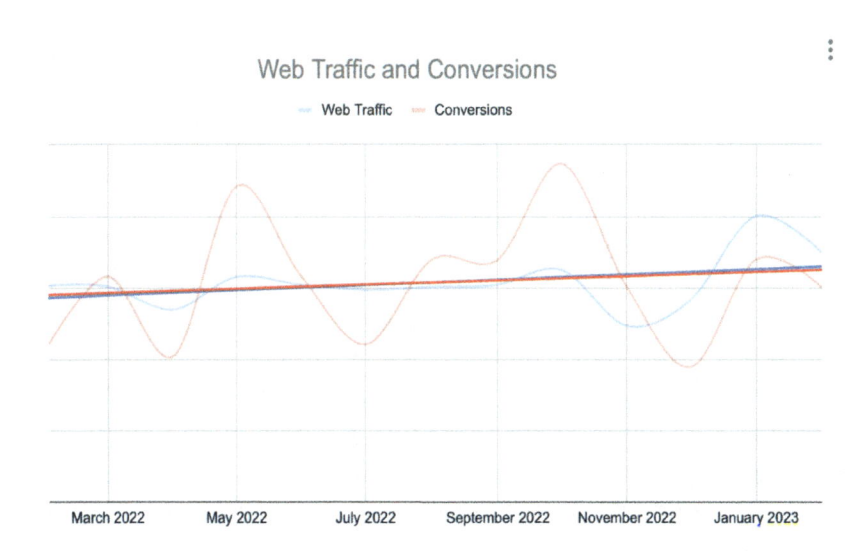

Conclusion

Flexibility in operations and marketing can be a critical factor in a practice's success. After fixing their branding and building a foundation, Mount Vernon Smile Design was able to have flexibility within their operations to allow the practice to test out different marketing strategies. Using what we learned, and staying flexible on the operations side, we were able to focus on hygiene and general new patients to fill up the hygiene schedule when that was needed. At other times, we have been focusing on emergencies and developing out more of the implant materials to generate more interest there as well.

From Dr. Whitney Forsythe

'My husband and I bought our practice in 2019 from a retiring doctor. While we had an established patient base, new patient numbers were low, hovering around 10-11/month. We knew growth would be a necessity if we were going to support two doctors.

After about eight months of running our own marketing program, we quickly realized our new patient numbers were stagnant. We needed support in order to fill a second doctor's schedule and add more hygiene days. Ryan and his team worked to revamp our website, utilizing Google analytics to improve our visibility. They took over our social media accounts, using a data-based approach to attract patients, while also providing us with in-house marketing ideas such as referral rewards and ways to grow our google review count.

Over the past few years, we have introduced multiple specialties into the practice including clear aligners, endo, and various surgeries. Using a marketing strategy focused on referrals, specialty deals, and emergency visits, we've grown our new patients from 10/month to an average of 35-40 as well as increased monthly production.'

Takeaways

- Rebranding is sometimes needed prior to starting marketing campaigns to ensure best results.
- Paralleling capacity to the right services and flexing marketing with the business allows for a laser focus on which lever to pull and when.
- Determining if marketing efforts are better optimized externally or internally is key to expanding services.

CHAPTER 3

Broad Smiles Pediatric Dentistry and Orthodontics

Locations - Lynn and Salem, Massachusetts
Doctors - 3
Annual Production - $2.5 Million

Practice Overview

Broad Smiles Pediatric Dentistry & Orthodontics is a multi-location pediatric practice with locations in Lynn and Salem Massachusetts. The practice focuses on pediatric dentistry with an emphasis on frenectomy, orthodontics, and specialty pediatric care. They are well-known in their area for frenectomy treatments and have a strong and reputable brand in the markets they serve.

Challenge and Growth Opportunity

Dr. Hubert Park, owner of Broad Smiles Pediatric Dentistry & Orthodontics, built his flagship location in Lynn, Massachusetts. The practice had a strong brand reputation in the area due to high quality care for infants and children as well as being regionally known for performing frenectomy procedures. When they opened their second location in Salem, we wanted to ensure this reputation and brand awareness not only transferred to the new location but was leveraged to quickly attain new patients in Salem. We also wanted to increase the number of higher value patients so we could continue to increase revenue even after we reached capacity for general new patients. This was the foundation of the marketing strategy we developed.

The Work

As we approached the new location for Salem, we first identified the marketing opportunities and priorities:

1. Utilize the existing brand awareness of Lynn and online market share.
2. Schedule new patients from Lynn to Salem if possible to quickly boost Salem.
3. Schedule all frenectomy appointments from Salem to Lynn to add revenue to Lynn.

Next, we also identified the challenges:

1. Increasing local website traffic and local conversions.
2. Expanding the online presence to Salem (Google Business Profile, Facebook)
3. Zeroing in on new patients under 2 years of age

We took a data-driven approach to address these challenges. Our initial efforts led to a significant increase in local organic traffic from 150 visits to over 400 visits a month. However, we realized that much of this traffic focused on teenager orthodontics, which did not align with their strategy of patient acquisition of children under two years old. While an Orthodontic start was a good hit of instant revenues, we actually didn't want to fill chair time with teenagers yet. A new patient under the age two actually leads to a higher lifetime patient value.

To address this, we made adjustments to target "baby's first dental visit." This change in focus led to an immediate increase in new patient numbers for the Salem location.

The Results

Within three months, the new patient flow at Salem had doubled, and after two years, the location saw an average of 50 new patients per month.

Results after shifting the SEO focus:

1. Increased localized web traffic to over 400 visits per month.

2. Boosted new patient numbers in the Salem location from 20 to 50 per month.

3. Both practices reached capacity for new patients, allowing for a shift in marketing focus to higher value treatments.

You will see in the attached chart that in March of 2022, Lynn reached max capacity and needed to decrease new patients in order to ensure they could see all current patients.

NP and Production

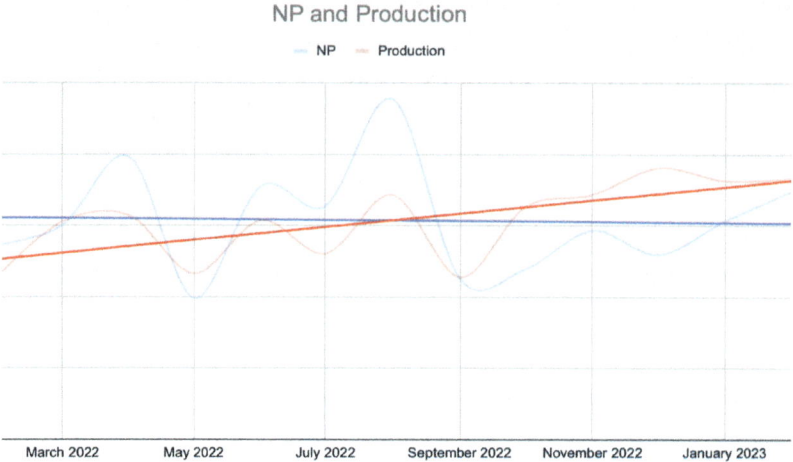

— NP — Production

March 2022 May 2022 July 2022 September 2022 November 2022 January 2023

During this time Salem's new patients increased and toward the end of 2022 and beginning of 2023 they reached capacity. Once this point occurred at Salem, new patient numbers decreased for both practices. We anticipated this occurring, which is why at the same time, we also invested in frenectomy, sedation and orthodontics marketing. As you can from the graph, even though new patient total numbers decreased, production still increased.

Conclusion

This case study highlights the importance of targeted marketing in helping practices grow and optimize new patient flow and production. By understanding the specific needs and goals of Broad Smiles Pediatric Dentistry & Orthodontics, we were able to tailor the marketing efforts to reach the right audience at the right time, driving new patient growth at Salem revenue for both practices after they reached capacity for new patients.

Takeaways:

- Identifying your ideal patient ensures marketing efforts are focused on the audience with the highest value return.
- Ensure marketing is empowering your short-term goal of new patients, while also considering a long-term approach of higher value patients. This allows you to easily evolve to continue increasing revenue once your office reaches capacity.

CHAPTER 4

Humlicek Family Dental

Location - Wichita, Kansas
Doctors - 1
Annual Production - $1.8 million

Practice Overview

Humlicek Family Dental is a general practice that focuses on cosmetic treatment such as clear aligners, whitening, and implants. The practice is owned by Dr. Ashley Humlicek, and focuses heavily on patient experience, brand awareness, and showcasing the unique differences from their competitors.

Challenge and Growth Opportunity

Dr. Ashley Humlicek is not your average dentist. As a competitive college swimmer, she has always attacked life with drive and a competitive nature. This approach to life is a large part of the driving force behind Humlicek Family Dental. Dr. Humlicek has created a unique approach to dentistry that is reflected in her practice's impressive results. This approach includes a focus on general dentistry that increases active patient count, but then leverages these numbers to add more cosmetic procedures. This accelerated growth has led to the practice's current capacity issue, and she is hoping to alleviate that in the next year as she builds a new larger space with 12 operatories.

The Work

When we first started working with Dr. Humlicek, our goal was to increase online market share for more new hygiene patients–the practice had availability to increase new patient flow. Our strategy was to build a strong brand around Dr. Humlicek, followed by increasing web traffic and Google reviews.

Our first step was rebranding the practice to represent Dr. Humlicek's vision. She wanted her brand tied closely to the city of Wichita and to feel warm and welcoming to patients. We used elements of the Wichita city flag as inspiration for the brand and the logo, including the colors and iconography. Next, we ensured images of Dr. Humlicek and her team were included in almost every marketing piece–and they had to be images that looked approachable and unposed. The practice is heavily focused on a comfortable and welcoming patient experience, so we wanted to ensure the photos and the overall brand reflected this feeling.

After the rebranding, which included a new website, new logo and internal branding elements, we began focusing on patient acquisition. We determined that her web traffic was including areas of Wichita that did not equate to new patients. For example, the website was receiving visits from the eastern part of the city, but new patients were all coming from the western half. We adjusted the Google ad strategy and targeting to focus on the areas where patients were converting at a higher rate. Using OpenDental to look at zip codes of new patients allowed for this research to be done easily.

After establishing consistent web traffic and high actual conversion rate, the practice began to reach capacity. At that point, we wanted to focus on ways to increase production that didn't require hygiene appointments. We then created an emergency dental campaign to increase demand on the doctor's schedule. This helped slightly, but then the ideas started coming that would be truly innovative.

Dr. Humlicek had an idea to attend a wedding fair in the area with the goal of increasing clear aligner and cosmetic cases. To prepare for the wedding fair, we worked with Dr. Humlicek to create a strategy that included items for her booth and an online marketing push. For the booth, she needed traditional items such as pull banners, tablecloth, signage, and items to give away. The primary message was centered around "A Timeline for Your Wedding Smile." She wanted to create a space that included clear messaging, showcased technology, and included special offers. Dr. Humlicek also brought her iTero scanner and performed scans on attendees at her booth.

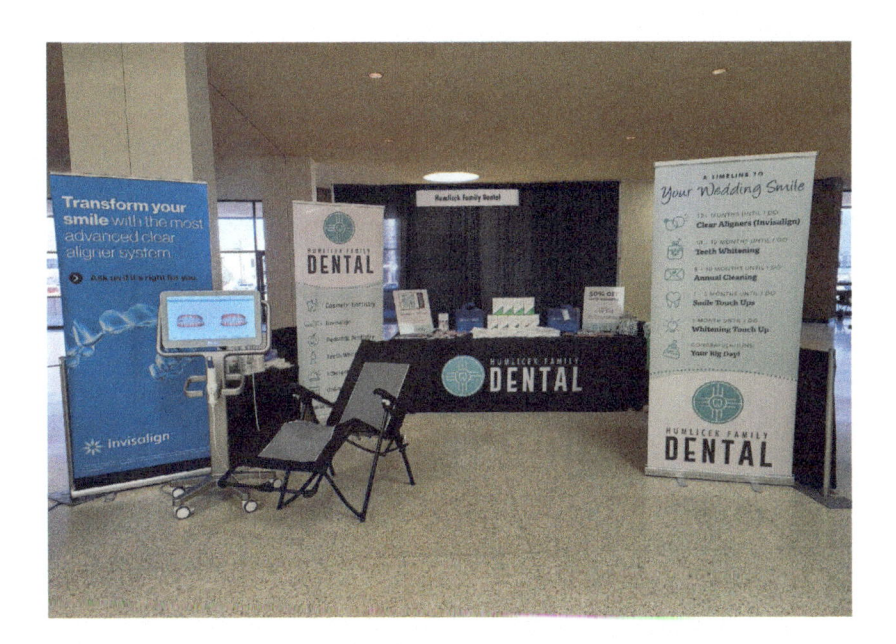

To complement the event on-site marketing we created an online strategy that included a landing page on the website, Google and Facebook Ads, and updated content on the "service" pages that were being showcased at the event. The ads were placed the week prior to the event and two weeks after. The ads featured services such as clear aligners and teeth whitening with the goal of showing up on searches from people who attended the event.

The Results

The results were amazing and really proved Dr. Humlicek was correct that this idea would be successful.

- Website traffic increased 258% the day of the event
- Total website traffic for the week after the event was up 26%
- 58 appointments were made the weekend of and the week after the event

Users	Sessions	Bounce Rate	Session Duration
423	**507**	**45.56%**	**1m 28s**
↑40.5%	↑33.4%	↑1.8%	↓20.3%

The day of the event

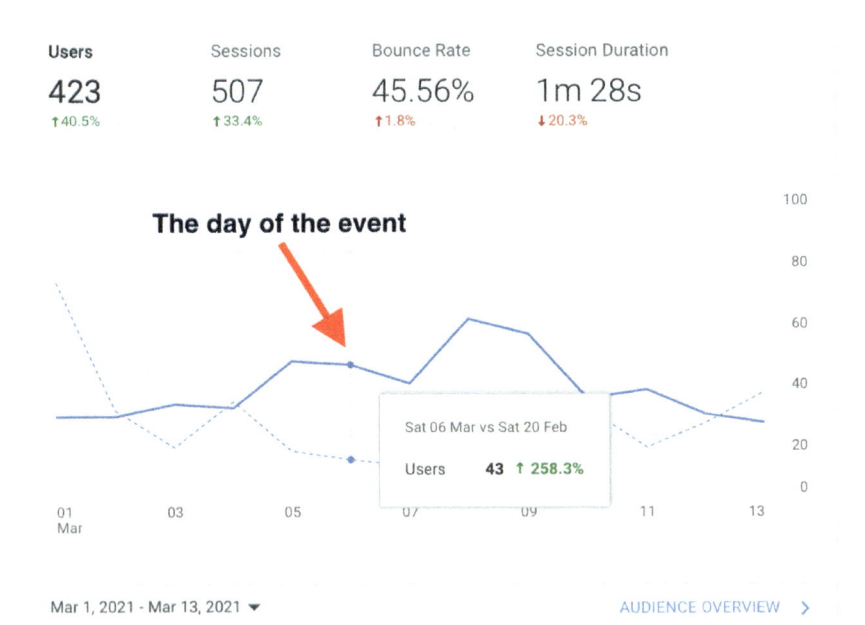

Sat 06 Mar vs Sat 20 Feb
Users 43 ↑ 258.3%

Mar 1, 2021 - Mar 13, 2021   AUDIENCE OVERVIEW >

Over the past year, Humlicek Family Dental has generated $1,839,576 in production and received 404 new patient visits. These impressive numbers are a testament to Dr. Humlicek's commitment to patient satisfaction and innovation. She and her team go above and beyond to ensure that each patient feels heard and cared for, which is why they have an average Google review rating of 4.9 out of 5 based on 430 reviews and a perfect Facebook review rating of 5 out of 5 based on 21 reviews.

The increase in her new patients, active patients, and revenue has enabled Dr. Humlicek to look to build a new practice that is much larger than her current space and will have an area focusing on a dental spa experience. This new practice will allow her to continue building her general patient flow, which is her bread and butter, but at the same time allow her to expand on her cosmetic services and be known in Wichita as the premier practice for cosmetic dentistry.

One of the key findings from our analysis, which is generally what we see in almost every scenario, is that web traffic and conversions generally leads to more production. The chart below confirms the trends.

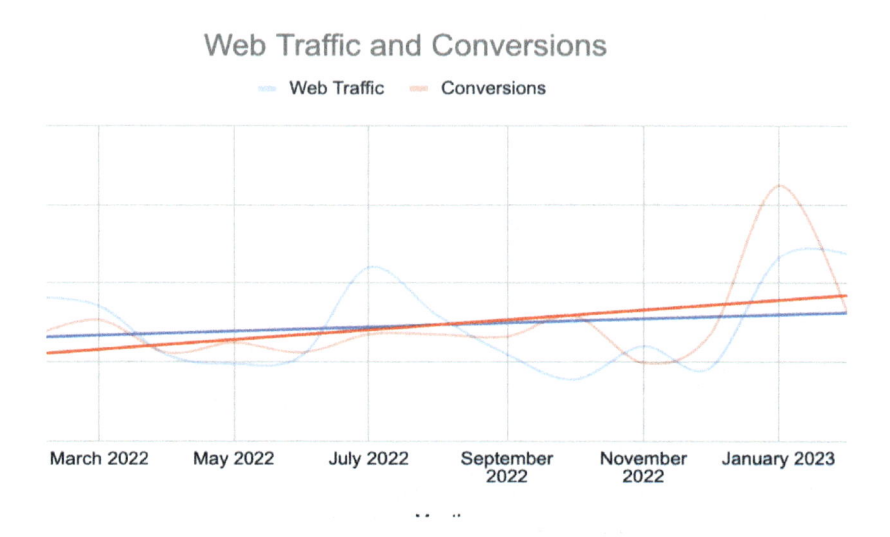

Web Traffic and Conversions

— Web Traffic   — Conversions

| March 2022 | May 2022 | July 2022 | September 2022 | November 2022 | January 2023 |

Humlicek Family Dental is a valuable case study for practices looking to optimize their online presence and thinking outside the typical marketing box. 58 Invisalign consult or start appointments from 1 marketing campaign could lead to almost a quarter-million dollars in revenue from one marketing push, not to mention the possible longer-term benefits of being known as the Invisalign dentist in Wichita.

Conclusion

With a smaller practice and limited capacity, it is important to find ways to increase production without having to increase overall new patient flow. Having a strong brand and online as your foundation will allow you to capitalize on marketing opportunities that are outside the box such as wedding fairs or more specialty services.

From Dr. Ashley Humlicek

'Buying a practice from a retiring doctor seemed ideal until I realized how often we were sending out sympathy cards to deceased patient's families. A dental practice tends to "age" with the doctor so we were desperately in need of younger patients that would be with us for years to come. Marketing allowed us to focus our efforts on our ideal avatar and grow the practice the way we wanted it to grow. After an influx in growth, we needed to create block scheduling to ensure we had space for the constant demand. Now after steady growth and systematic scheduling, we are able to do more targeted marketing for high dollar procedures like implants, cosmetic dentistry and Invisalign. Marketing has allowed us to build our ideal practice for a specific snapshot in time and it changes as we continue to evolve.'

Takeaways:

- Building your brand is an important first step to any successful practice
- Unique marketing opportunities in the community can spike web traffic and lead to huge revenue afterwards
- If you are planning on doing any physical expansion, make sure your web traffic and market share is growing to fill up these operatories once completed

CHAPTER 5

Finger Lakes Dental Care

Location - Western New York State (5 locations)
Doctors - 11
Annual Production - $15+ million

Practice Overview

Finger Lakes Dental Care is a five-location practice located in west New York owned by Dr. Jason Tanoory. The practices focus on general dentistry, emergency services, implants, oral surgery, sedation and clear aligners. They are well-known in their rural area for a teamwork atmosphere and from Dr. Tanoory's involvement in the community over the past decades.

Challenge and Growth Opportunity

When we started working with Finger Lakes, they had four locations and a fifth one on the way. Our goal was to create an online marketing strategy where all the locations lived under one brand and one website but allowed for each location to also have separate marketing strategies based upon operational and location needs. At the time their marketing strategy did include one brand and one website, but the setup and user experience did not allow for the ideal individual optimization.

The Work

We identified an opportunity early on that would create a large online market share based upon the locations of each practice. This would then give more opportunities for one of their locations to show up on organic search results and paid ads. The Google map shows where each of their locations are in relation to each other.

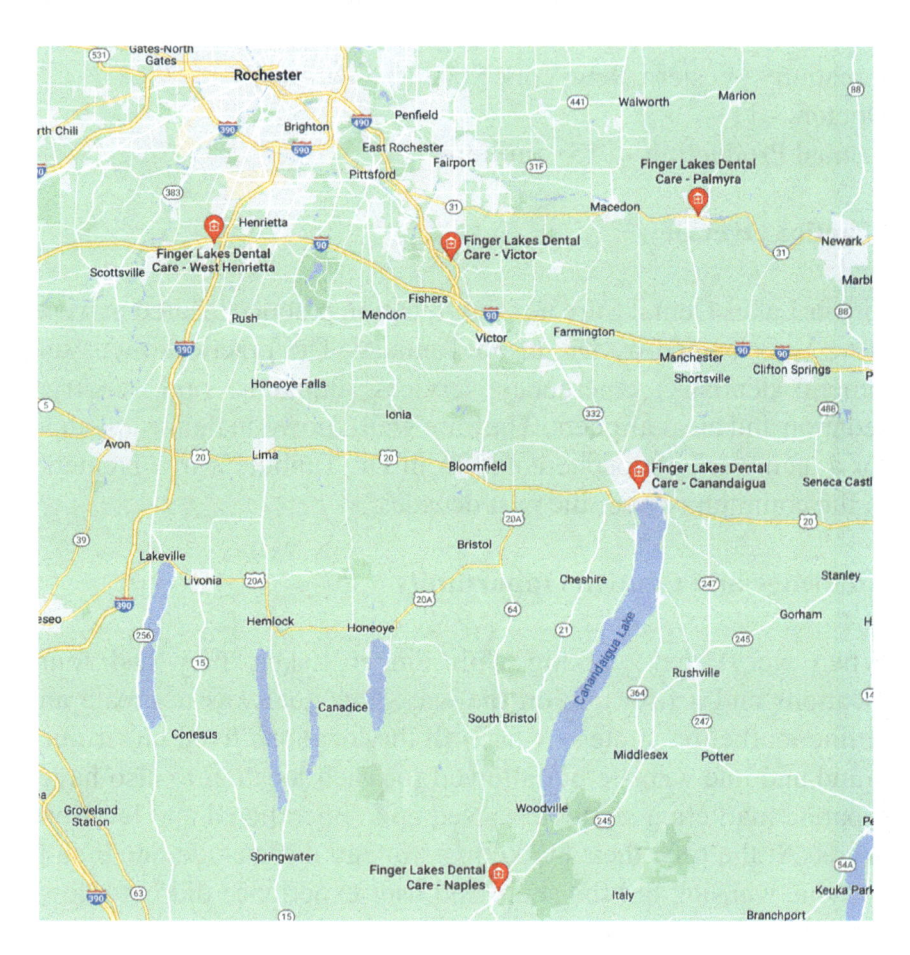

In the next map you can see our strategy of overlapping online market share leading to a possible new patient searching for a dentist and two of the Finger Lakes locations showing up on a search result.

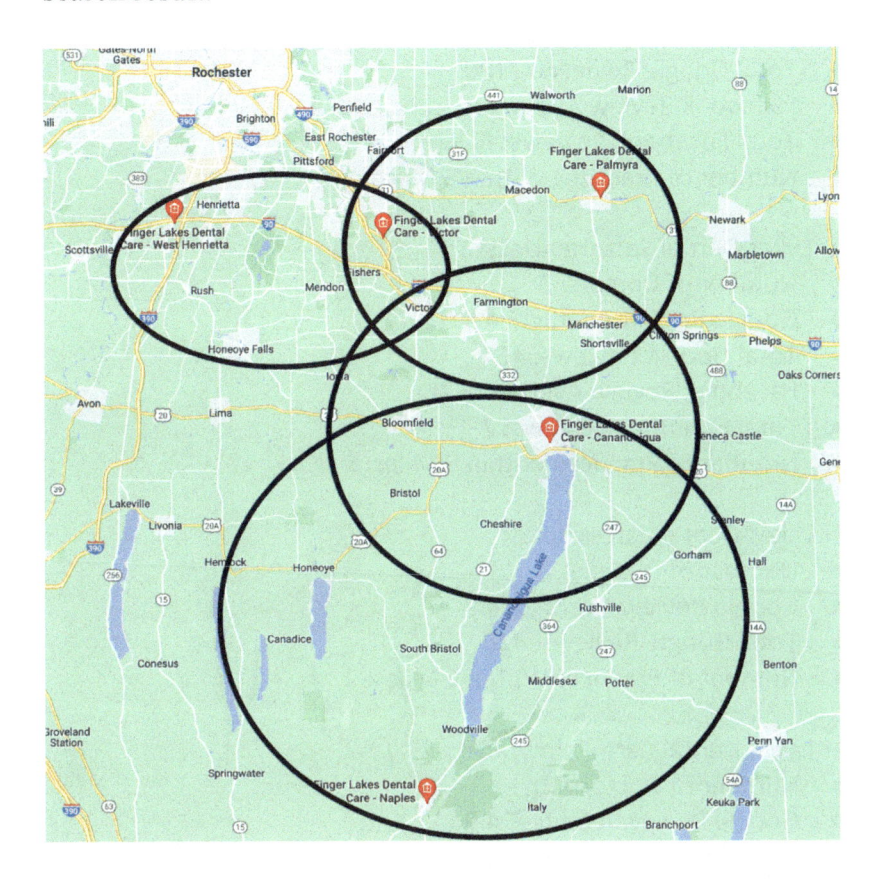

Location Overviews

Finger Lakes Dental Care-Canandaigua (Flagship)

- Number of Doctors: 7
- Google Review Average: 4.9
- Total Google Reviews: 2100
- Facebook Review Average: 5
- Total Facebook Reviews: 6
- Number of Practices Within 5 Miles: 4

Finger Lakes Dental Care-Henrietta
- Number of Doctors: 3
- Google Review Average: 4.9
- Total Google Reviews: 464
- Facebook Review Average: 5.0
- Total Facebook Reviews: 2
- Number of Practices Within 5 Miles: 5

Finger Lakes Dental Care-Naples:
- Number of Doctors: 2
- Google Review Average: 4.9
- Total Google Reviews: 428
- Number of Practices Within 5 Miles: 2

Finger Lakes Dental Care-Palmyra:
- Number of Doctors: 2
- Google Review Average: 4.9
- Total Google Reviews: 585
- Number of Practices Within 5 Miles: 2

Finger Lakes Dental Care-Victor:

- Number of Doctors: 2
- Google Review Average: 4.9
- Total Google Reviews: 154
- Number of Practices Within 5 Miles: 5

We created one website that a user could easily navigate to from the homepage and see all the locations. Each location page on the master website encompassed the critical information a patient would want to know about a specific location of Finger Lakes Dental Care. These expanded location pages also allowed for each practice location to showcase its own brand and unique selling points. This approach also allowed for Google to recognize one overall Finger Lakes Dental as well as the separate locations. This expanded search results significantly and allowed for the practice to come up as Finger Lakes Dental if the user wasn't sure of the location they were wanting to visit, and for each location to show up separately for users who did know the location they wanted to visit.

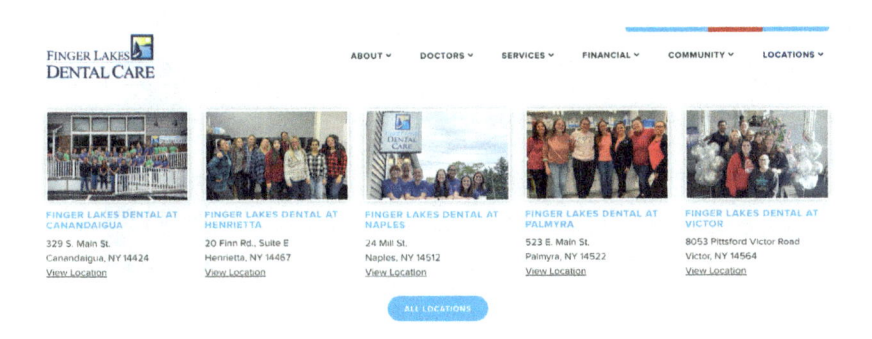

Finger Lakes Dental Care
https://fingerlakesdental.com

Finger Lakes Dental Care - 5 Locations Across New York ...
Finger Lakes Dental Care offers superior dental care with five convenient locations across New York. Schedule your dentist appointment today.
Locations · Finger Lakes Dental at Palmyra · Finger Lakes Dental at Canandaigua

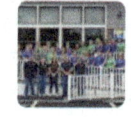

Finger Lakes Dental Care
https://fingerlakesdental.com › locations

5 Locations Across New York
Finger Lakes Dental at Canandaigua. 329 S. Main St. Canandaigua, NY 14424. View Map · (585) 394-1930 ; Finger Lakes Dental at Henrietta. 20 Finn Rd., Suite E

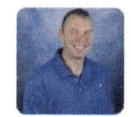

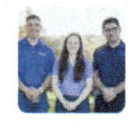

Finger Lakes Dental Care
https://fingerlakesdental.com › locations › palmyra

Finger Lakes Dental at Palmyra, NY
The Palmyra, NY dentist office of Finger Lakes Dental offers comprehensive dental services to patients. Schedule your appointment today.

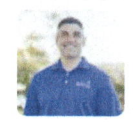

Finger Lakes Dental Care
https://fingerlakesdental.com › locations › canandaigua

Finger Lakes Dental at Canandaigua
Dentist office in Canandaigua, NY offering general dentistry, a pediatric dentist, and oral surgeon. Call Finger Lakes Dental Canandaigua.

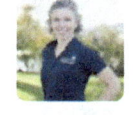

Finger Lakes Dental Care
https://fingerlakesdental.com › financial

Affordable Dental Care - Finger Lakes Dental - New York
Locations ; Finger Lakes Dental at Canandaigua. 329 S. Main St. Canandaigua, NY 14424. (585) 394-1930 ; Finger Lakes Dental at Henrietta. 20 Finn Rd., Suite E

Our online marketing strategy includes optimization for the overall brand and website–since each location falls under the Finger Lakes Dental Care brand name, using a strategy around that name propels and supports all offices across the practice. The website houses all information for the overall Finger Lakes Dental Care brand and is flexible enough to dive into information specific to a single practice only such as the staff and doctors, hours, and other information that is local to that location. More specifically, we can also optimize the local practice pages based upon competitors and the market.

The user also has the opportunity to schedule online or to learn more specifics on each location. Users can also learn about career opportunities and working for Finger Lakes Dental. On the individual location pages, we can also detail information about the location

The Results

The results of this strategy allowed the practice to grow online market share and increase overall website traffic from April 2022 to April 2023 by 19 percent. They currently receive an average of 5,200 web visits a month.

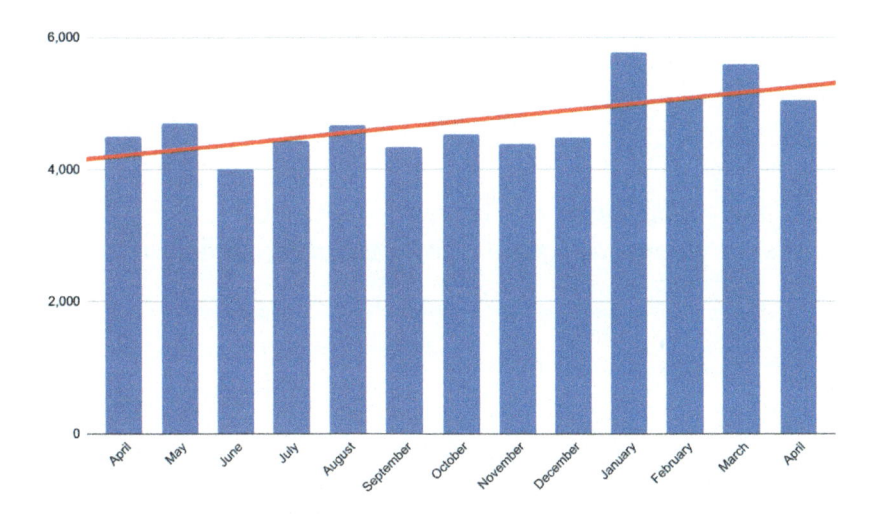

53

Conclusion

Large multi-location practices such as Finger Lakes Dental Care should use their size and reach to leverage their overall brand but also should have the ability to individually focus on each location and their specific marketing and operational needs. When you build the right scaffolding to take advantage of both your size, as well as individual locations, you can gain market share quickly.

Amy Ells, Chief Operating Officer

"We want people to know who we are and what we believe in. As we expand into new towns, we have been able to link our locations together online and inspire trust in the new office based on the reputation of our established offices. We have been able to add specialists to our team and we have been able to target people looking for these specialized services.

Without marketing all of our offices together, but separately, we wouldn't see the continued growth we have had year over year."

Takeaways:

- Multiple-location practices can extend market share by connecting all their website across a common name, while keeping sites local for Search-Engine Optimization
- Creating a corporate web structure also allows team members and patients to see the core values that the entire organization believes in, while increasing recruitment of new team members
- Branding is extremely important in attracting and retaining high quality talent

CHAPTER 6

Markowitz Family Dental

Locations - Massachusetts (6 locations)
Doctors - 19
Annual Production - $20+ million

Practice Overview

Markowitz Family Dental (MFD) Dental is a group practice located in Massachusetts owned by Dr. Steve Markowitz. The practice was started by his father and Dr. Steve has not only continued the legacy but grown it exponentially after taking over management of the practices while still a dental student. The growing company now consists of six locations, focusing on general dentistry, implants and emergency care. Each practice is named based upon the community they are located in but branded similarly with logo and colors.

Challenge and Growth Opportunity

In this case study we will examine a large multi-location practice similar to Finger Lakes Dental Care, but that does not share the same name–rather each location has a separate name related to the community of the practice. When we first started with Dr. Markowitz, MFD owned three locations. Each practice was named differently but were branded similarly. Instead of renaming all the practices and bringing them under one name we chose to continue with their individual names, while trying to unify the branding and color schemes. I will detail how we created a plan that optimized the market share of each location to benefit all of the locations.

Since each location has a separate website, it gives us full control over optimizing each practice individually. Unlike Finger Lakes Dental Care where a website user can navigate and find the location most convenient for them, users of MFD practices only can choose that location on the website. Knowing this we wanted to build authority and market share as quickly as possible for the three practices that we started with.

Location Overviews

Leominster Family Dentists (Flagship)
- Number of Doctors: 9
- Google Review Average: 4.9
- Total Google Reviews: 829
- Facebook Review Average: 4.9
- Total Facebook Reviews: 346
- Number of Practices Within 5 Miles: 7

Drum Hill Dental
- Number of Doctors: 4
- Google Review Average: 4.9
- Total Google Reviews: 434
- Facebook Review Average: 5
- Total Facebook Reviews: 98
- Number of Practices Within 5 Miles: 11

Nashoba Family Dentists
- Number of Doctors: 7
- Google Review Average: 4.9
- Total Google Reviews: 517
- Facebook Review Average: 5.0

- Total Facebook Reviews: 64
- Number of Practices Within 5 Miles: 9

Maynard Family Dentists
- Number of Doctors: 2
- Google Review Average: 4.9
- Total Google Reviews: 115
- Facebook Review Average: 5
- Total Facebook Reviews: 14
- Number of Practices Within 5 Miles: 7

Lakeview Family Dentists
- Number of Doctors: 5
- Google Review Average: 4.9
- Total Google Reviews: 195
- Facebook Review Average: 5
- Total Facebook Reviews: 21
- Number of Practices Within 5 Miles: 14

Century Family Dental
- Number of Doctors: 1
- Google Review Average: 5
- Total Google Reviews: 29
- Facebook Review Average: x
- Total Facebook Reviews: x
- Number of Practices Within 5 Miles: 9

Each practice is branded similarly but named differently. Included are three of the practice's logos.

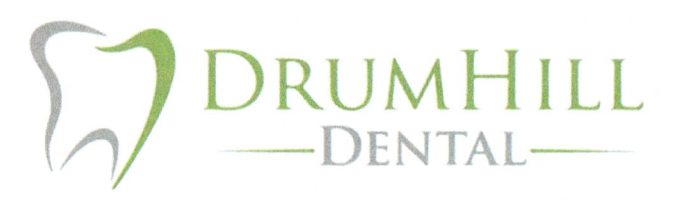

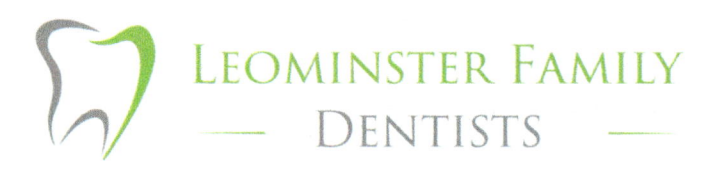

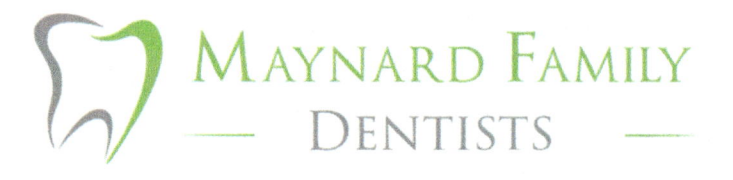

Included is a before and after example of the Leominster practice prior to the brand unification and new website.

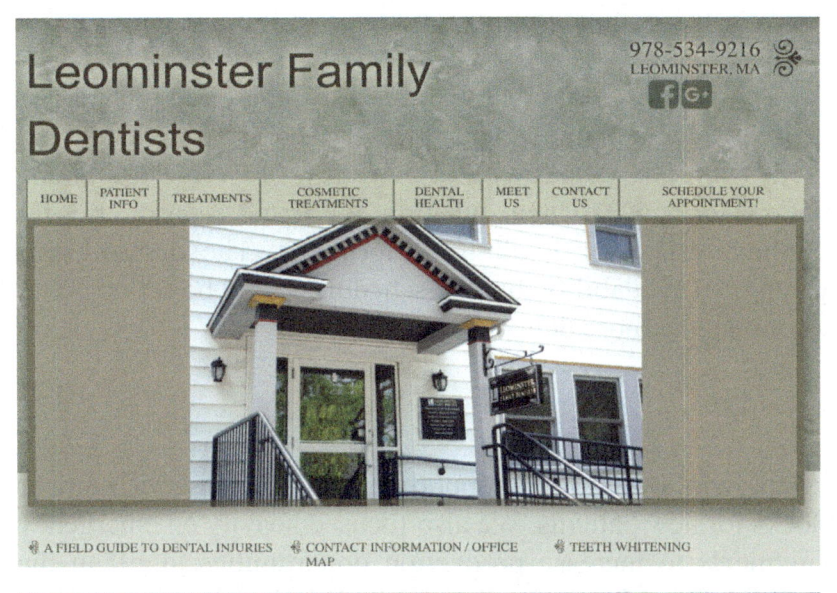

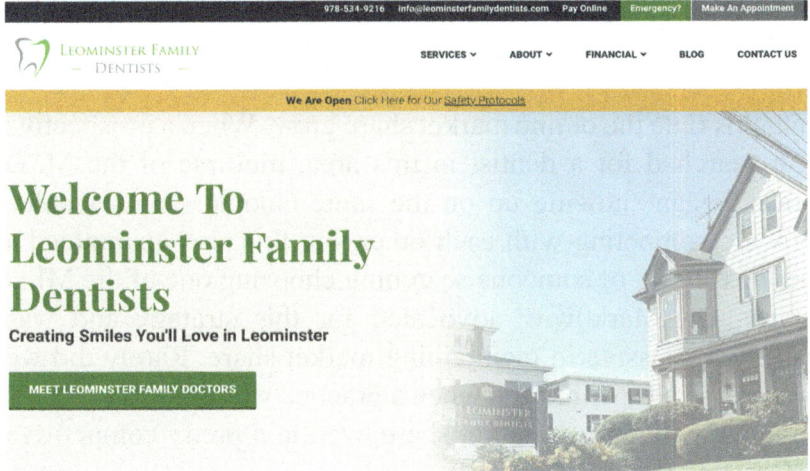

The Work

We first identified the specific strategy for each location. For example, Leominster Family Dentists was nearly at capacity, so we looked at increasing emergency appointments to increase revenue. Whereas Drum Hill Dental was in a crowded market and had room to grow their new patient base. For Drum Hill, we focused on the competitors in the area and how to gain market share.

Once we created and implemented the strategy for each location, I worked with Dr. Markowitz to ensure we were optimizing operations for new patient acquisition. We found opportunities for scheduling efficiency at all three locations. The demand was outpacing the availability, but the schedules could be set up better to accommodate more demand.

The Results

Dr. Markowitz's team found opportunities to increase the number of blocks for new patients. We also focused heavily on emergency appointments to increase production opportunities to fill in the gaps that inevitably occurred in the schedule due to same day cancellations.

During this time the online market share grew. When a prospective patient searched for a dentist in this area, multiple of the MFD practices began showing up on the same Google search results. They were competing with each other, but this also guaranteed a higher possibility of someone searching choosing one of the MFD practices. Dr. Markowitz advocated for this strategy and was purposely aggressive in maintaining market share. Rarely did we ever decrease ad spend, even when a practice was at capacity. This ensured we maintained market share even in a pretty competitive East Coast market.

In 2022, MFD began acquiring additional practices. Our strategy was to continue with what worked with the first three practices. We would analyze the area and choose a name for the practice that had local value to the residents but also SEO value. The next two practices added were Lakeview Family Dentist and Maynard Family Dentist. We approached each new practice with an aggressive marketing strategy to increase market share and online visibility as quickly as possible. At the same, operationally each practice was set up to maximize online conversions and ensure scheduling was optimized.

The attached graph shows web traffic, new patients and production for Maynard. You will see the accelerated growth based upon the increase in web traffic. The increase in new patients and production didn't occur until two months after the opening of Maynard when it moved to a new location with more physical visibility.

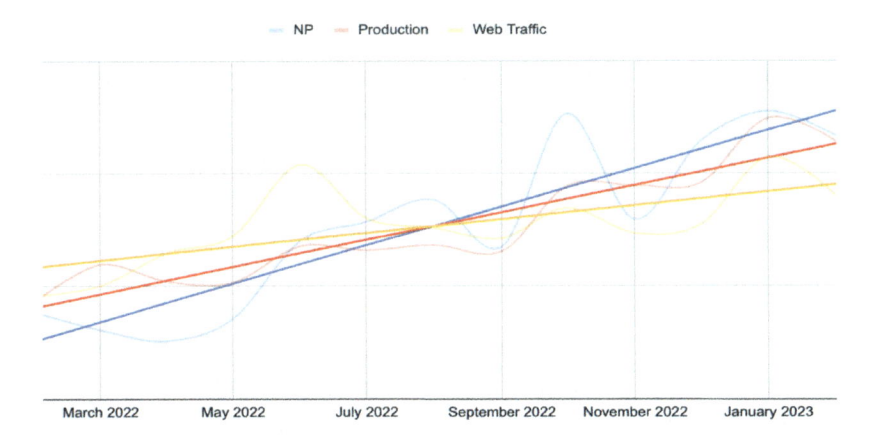

Like Maynard, the next attached chart for Lakeview shows the same growth but in this case web traffic, new patients and production are nearly identical.

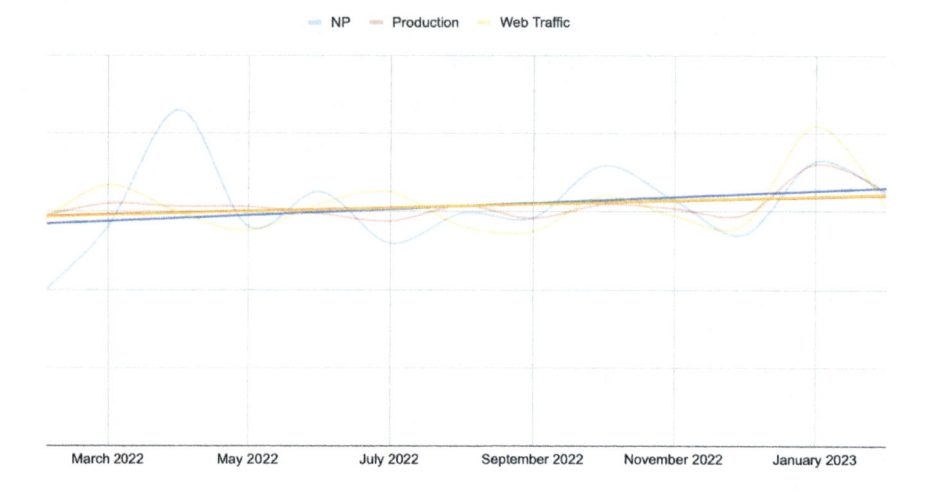

Conclusion

Part of MFD Dental's success was naming each practice with a local tie to the community. This typically isn't recommended in a multi-location group, but in this case we were able to take advantage of those local ties, optimize each practice individually and work together to ensure success across all of their locations.

From an Operations standpoint, Dr. Markowitz has done many things that ensured the practices grew. Number one was being ready with staffing to optimize the locations. This mean hiring more hygienists, assistants and doctors to be ready for this growth. Secondly was block scheduling, and making sure that when marketing occurred, there were blocks to allow for those patients to schedule.

However, the final and most important piece is an insane focus on the patient experience. Team members are given budgets each week to create an amazing experience for a patient. If a patient talked about a book with a team member, the practice would go on Amazon.com and send the patient a book as a gift with a note. This unique approach to creating a fantastic experience is what has allowed MFD practices to grow at a logarithmic scale.

From Dr. Steve Markowitz

'In every successful dental practice, it is essential to understand how all departments intertwine and support one another to create our desired outcomes. There is none, in my opinion, that have a greater connection and dependency than marketing and operations. Marketing is the mouth that feeds the operation of the business, operations must understand the messaging and volume that marketing is looking to capture or both departments will not be optimized or efficient.

In a time when the business of dentistry is becoming most challenging and every expense line item is being stretched, understanding the codependency of marketing and operational efficiency has been a driver of our double-digit YoY revenue growth in all of our practice locations. This has been through systemizing operational capacity, understanding availability for new patients and their impact on revenue, and learning how to best capture our created demand.'

Takeaways:
- Being prepared for growth with hiring is of utmost importance
- Creating fantastic patient experience will lead to better return-on-investment for marketing dollars
- Some multiple location groups will be extremely successful when they brand individually to the local neighborhood or city, even at the risk of competing with each other for market share

CHAPTER 7

Summit Family Dentistry

Location - Denver, North Carolina
Doctors - 3
Annual Production - $3.2 Million

Practice Overview

Summit Family Dentistry is a single location practice located in Denver, North Carolina. The practice is owned by Dr. Andy Pernell and focuses on general and emergency dentistry. After bringing in one associate in 2021, the practice now has added a third doctor to continue growing.

Challenge and Growth Opportunity

This case study highlights the results of combining the right marketing with the right demographic with the right operations to handle growth. When I started working with the practice, Dr. Pernell was the only provider and was averaging around 60 new patients per month. The practice had a capacity issue and was booking new patients through hygiene out nearly two months. Dr. Pernell was starting to get burnt out and was stressed because he couldn't fit emergencies into his schedule quickly enough. This was even stressing out the team, as they neared burnout.

The Work

The first step for the practice was to on-board an Associate Dentist who could help handle the growth. With about 8 months of recruitment and planning, he finally hired his first associate. This process included a complete onboarding process, weekly and monthly check-ins that ensured that both doctors were treatment planning the same way and presenting information in the same fashion. With this doctor in place, we were then able to turn on the marketing machine.

Our first goal was to increase market share and brand awareness around his city of Denver, NC. While spending money on brand awareness, and not direct call-to-actions, might seem wasteful, it means that all future marketing dollars are actually more impactful. So we spent months building branding around town, and helping to make sure people just knew about Summit Family Dentistry.

We knew it was important in the community that patients felt connected to the practice. We built a website that showcased the brand, office, Dr. Pernell and team. Showcasing photos of his team and the doctor in the office would help create that connection. While we created the website, we also increased internal marketing by creating branded brochures, patient gifts, shirts, signage, and other items within the office. Included is an example of their core value poster.

SUMMIT FAMILY DENTISTRY

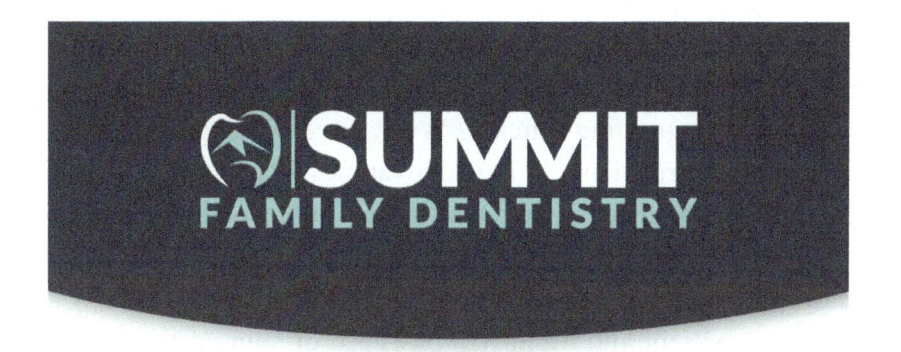

CORE VALUES

Our Core Values are what drives us in all of our actions and decision making in the office. These are simple and straightforward and what distinguishes our office from any other dental office. Lean on these values, always come back to them for reference if needed. Use them for open communication with each other. To help others when they are down, to hold others accountable, to make our work environment awesome. Thank you all!

AMAZING PATIENT EXPERIENCE
Our Goal is to exceed the expectations of each one of our patients, and we strive to do this with every patient, no matter what the circumstance.

PROFESSIONAL EXCELLENCE
We are driven by our ethics and morals as we strive to always do the right thing. We are respectful, helpful, and polished.

TEAM PLAYER
We understand and realize that we are all working together to provide an awesome experience for our patients and happy, healthy work environment for each other. Be there for one another, be selfless.

THE GOLDEN RULE
Treat others the way you wish to be treated. Be compassionate, caring, respectful, humble. Always do the right thing.

MISSION
Our mission is to strive to give each patient that walks through our doors a great experience from beginning to end and have fun doing it along the way.

VISION
Our vision is to change people's perception of the dentist for the better and continue to grow our influence on those we serve.

With the website complete and internal branding under way, we then created a postcard campaign to increase awareness. The postcards were mailed to newly built neighborhoods and a retirement community nearby. The town of Denver is near Charlotte and is growing quickly. We wanted to ensure we were reaching all new residents to create awareness that the practice is the premier dental office in the Denver area and reach families. We also sent postcards to the retirement residents. This was done to increase patients in the 55+ demographic. This demographic is a higher value patient and often will pay cash or sign up for the in-office savings plan.

These postcards included the amount of Google reviews, photos of the doctor and information on the saving plan.

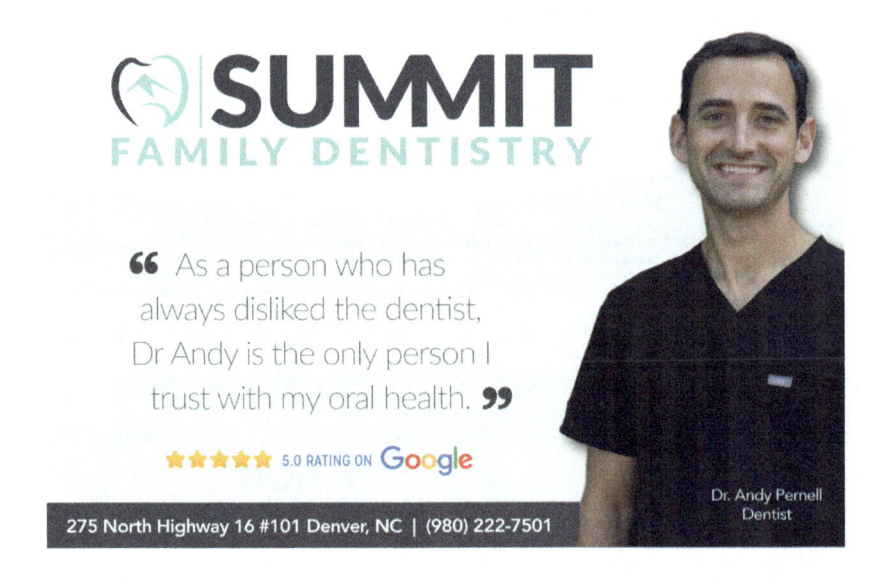

SUMMIT
FAMILY DENTISTRY

❝ As a person who has always disliked the dentist, Dr Andy is the only person I trust with my oral health. ❞

★★★★★ 5.0 RATING ON Google

275 North Highway 16 #101 Denver, NC | (980) 222-7501

Dr. Andy Pernell
Dentist

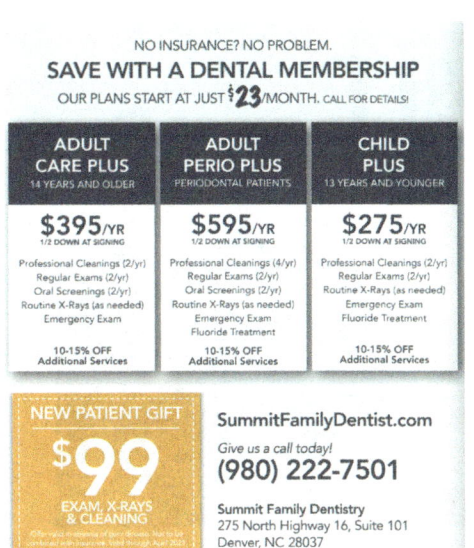

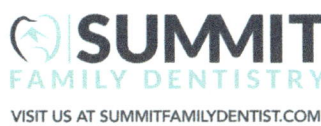

The Results

With all three marketing areas in place (online, internal and external) we began to see an increase in online market share. The practice quickly moved in the top three in visibility and Google rankings. With this increase in brand awareness and online presence, Dr. Pernell began to plot his next move, expanding the practice and hiring an additional associate doctor. Based upon the demand we were seeing through the website and in hygiene capacity, we predicted he would be able to hire another associate and fill the schedule quickly. To ensure this we increased Google Ads and sent another round of postcards. This time the postcards focused on all doctors and emergencies as well as the savings plan.

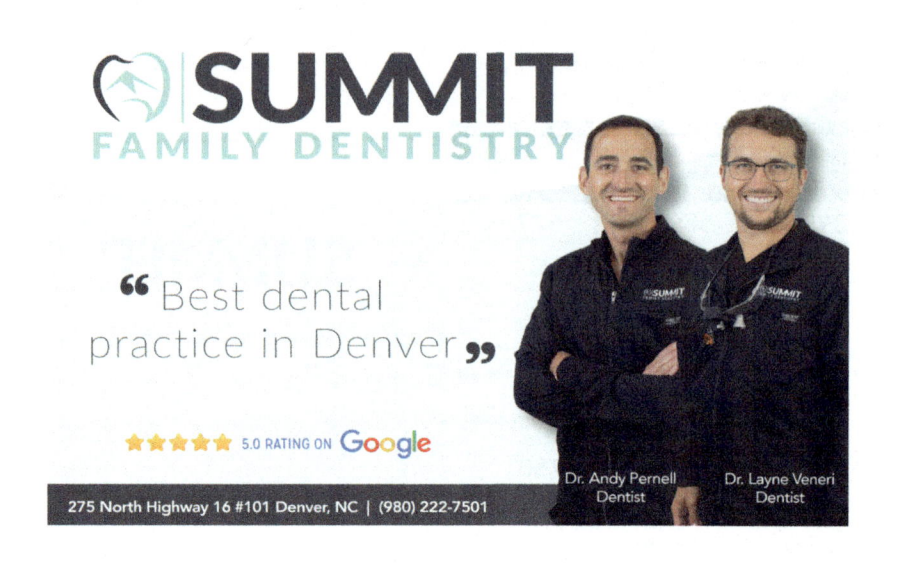

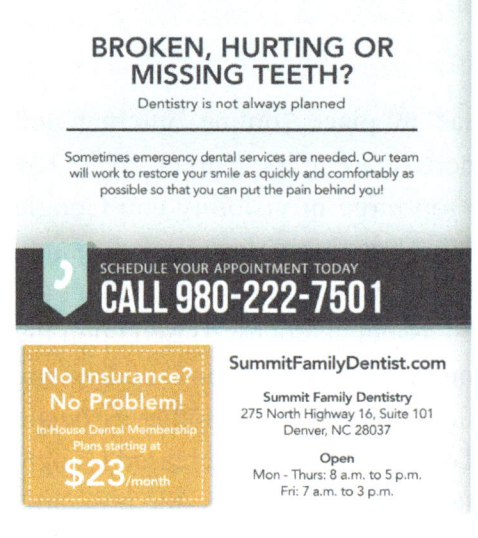

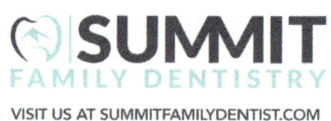

The practice grew quickly after these marketing efforts. New patients increased to an average of 90 and production doubled. The primary factor for capitalizing on the marketing success was the operations of the practice. Dr. Pernell and his office manager implemented systems to ensure marketing conversions resulted in actual new patients. They consistently answered over 85% of their calls. **This is the lead KPI along with website conversions.** The attached graph shows correlation between conversions, inbound calls and production. You can see the trendlines are nearly identical.

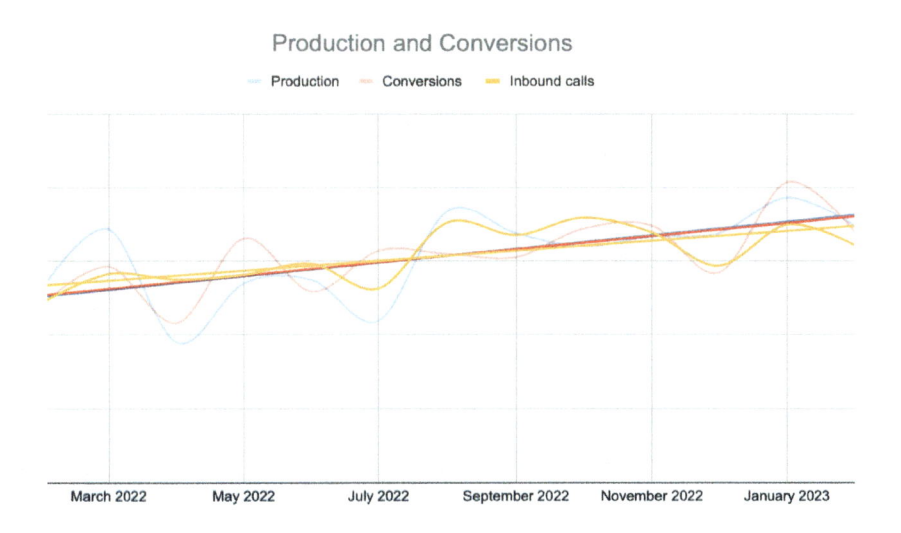

Production and Conversions

— Production   — Conversions   — Inbound calls

March 2022   May 2022   July 2022   September 2022   November 2022   January 2023

Conclusion

Summit Family Dentistry now has a space twice as large as it occupied just two years ago. The new patient demand continues to be strong, allowing Dr. Pernell to expand the practice's services into more specialties such as wisdom teeth extractions, implants and cosmetic dentistry. The combination between online, internal and external marketing created a strong brand awareness within the community and a large online market share.

From Dr. Andrew Pernell

"As our organization has grown, marketing continues to be one of the most important components of our operations. Understanding

our marketing data metrics, such as patient phone calls, conversions, and site traffic against market standards allows us to accurately forecast our monthly demand and revenue and run consistent operations month after month. Furthermore, by tracking this information we now react proactively versus reactively to an ever-changing market."

> Takeaways:
> - Bringing on an Associate Doctor can be one of the most important decisions for growth
> - Watching phone call answer rate and web traffic, you can prepare for growth and expansion
> - Once capacity is achieved, then specialization into high-value procedures can accelerate the growth of the practice

CHAPTER 8

Moorehead Family Dentistry

Location - Cincinnati, Ohio (3 locations)
Doctors - 5
Annual Production - $5+ Million

Practice Overview

Moorehead Family Dentistry is a multi-location practice in Cincinnati, Ohio. They have three locations and are owned by Dr. Doug Moorehead. All three locations and the associate doctors focus on general dentistry, while Dr. Moorehead focuses on surgical procedures and sedation dentistry.

Challenge and Growth Opportunity

This case study shows the importance of brand recognition and online scheduling. When we started working with Dr. Moorehead and his three locations had a large active patient base, but also had some room for growth.

The Work

We found that specifically, each location of Moorehead Family Dentistry needed an individual marketing strategy within the larger strategy that covers the Moorehead brand. Our goal with their online strategy was to increase visibility and market share across the brand as well as branded searches. The practice had strong web traffic to begin with. When we built the website, we wanted to capitalize on their strong foundation, but then cater to the localized searches as well. We were quickly able to remove web traffic that was not local and low value. We then focused on emergency patients, this allowed any of the locations that were at hygiene capacity to increase production.

As market share and web traffic increased for general and emergency services, we then moved to focusing on sedation dentistry. This process allowed the practice to grow production per patient even more without having to increase total new patients through hygiene.

The image below showcases new patients, sedation and all three of their locations.

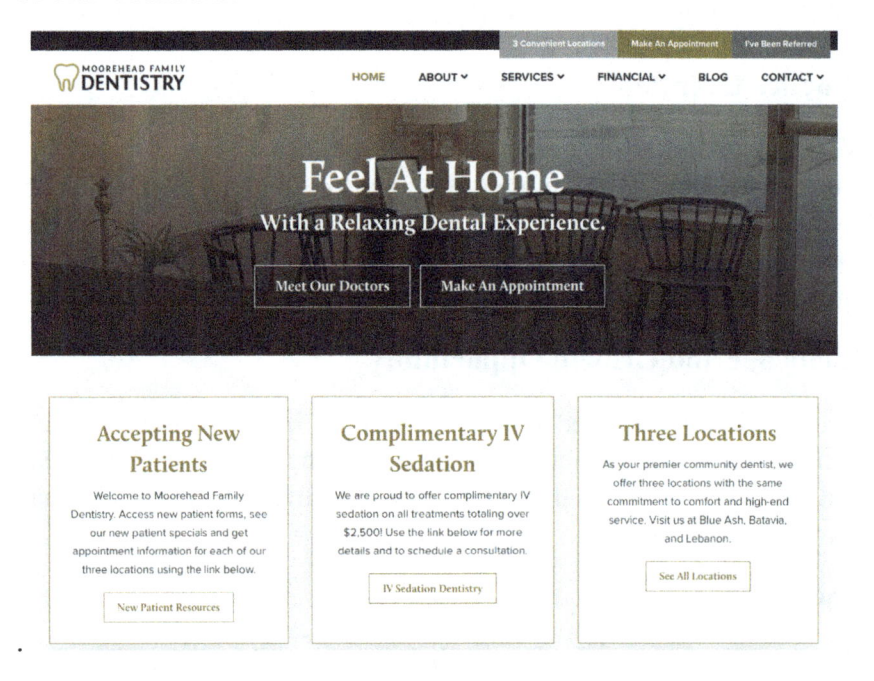

This image shows the different services the practice offers, including their focus services such as IV sedation, clear aligners, etc.

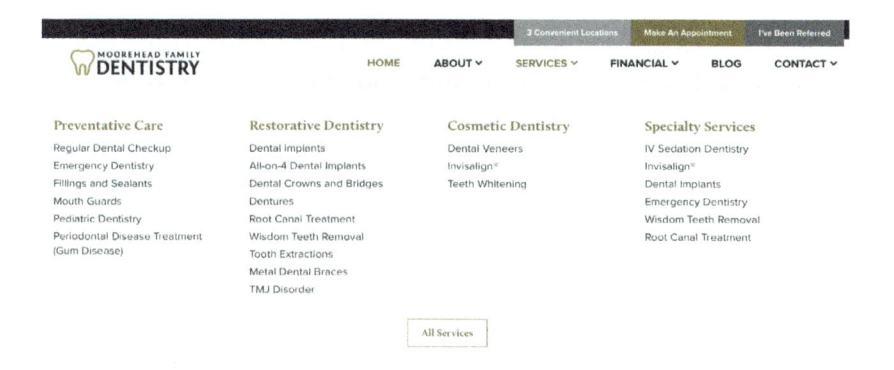

To ensure we were maximizing each location's potential, we were especially nimble with their Google ad campaigns. We would focus on general hygiene patients at a location that needed them and then focus on emergency patients and higher value services at locations that were at capacity. In Morehead's case we didn't need to increase web traffic as much as refine it to get higher production patients.

The attached graph shows the correlation between web traffic, conversions and production. You will see web traffic and conversions do increase but more importantly production increases as we focused on higher production marketing.

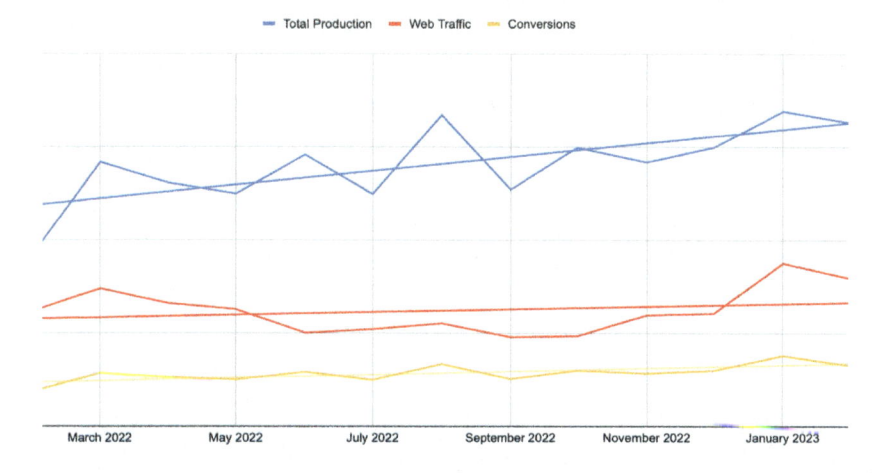

Perhaps the biggest operational key to their growth was the addition and success of online scheduling. When we found the

75

percent of clicks and calls moving in the afternoon and overnight hours, the practice moved to optimize the online scheduling. This led to more new patients scheduling, filling the gaps that are typically left open in practices that do not optimize their schedule.

This rush of new patients actually created a pinch in the hygiene scheduling, as they started to book out too far into the future. The dentists didn't get the chance to diagnose and treat the dental disease. Overall, this led to lower production numbers on the dental side, but very high production on the hygiene side. Dr. Moorehead and his team then came up with a better system to accelerate patients seen in a quicker time frame- letting new patients come in on the doctor's side of the practice.

They started to see all new patients on the doctor side of the practice for radiographs and an exam, and then reschedule later for their hygiene cleaning. This is a common theme among some practices but was new for Dr. Moorehead. This created confusion for some patients as they expected to be seen in hygiene for a cleaning on their first appointment. While some patients were surprised by the new system, the team worked diligently to communicate how the appointment would go. Phil Michael, Chief Operating Officer of Moorehead Family Dentistry, worked to make sure that each scheduler had a script to discuss this system with new patients, as well as details about this new system in their online scheduling portal. Phil pointed out that, "Setting the proper expectations to the patient was key in this success throughout the initial patient touch points. This allowed the doctor to diagnose restorative treatment sooner than had we waited on the patient coming in for their hygiene appointment, booking months out, or losing that patient altogether as they desired to be seen sooner."

The Results

By shifting the new patient appointment to the doctor side of the practice, they were able to balance the popularity of the hygiene appointment, with the need to fill the dentist's schedules quicker than previously anticipated.

Overall, the marketing of the practice was able to generate many new patients and increase market share, however it was through the operations of the practice that they were able to take advantage of that market share to translate that into revenue growth.

From Phil Michael- COO

"As a growing three-location practice in the suburbs of Cincinnati, OH, we looked to focus our marketing directly to new potential patients and establish branding throughout the city. We found that coordinating the marketing strategy with our operations was key in this strategy's success. To firmly establish our branding in the city, we relied on our paid marketing and optimized organic search results to drive prospective patients to our Google reviews. By incentivizing our clinical team to promote getting reviews and unifying the marketing efforts to drive new patients to those reviews, we found two major successes. Not only did our brand recognition increase in the city, but the new patients coming in were trusting us more from the start and also better represented the same value set as our previous patients who left 5-star reviews.

In regard to operations, our practice has always subscribed to the method of removing barriers for patients trying to schedule new patient appointments. By learning how many of our marketing conversions came after hours, we decided to provide online scheduling options and after-hours phone response to new patients to better convert those after-hours inquiries to new appointments. It also influenced our decision to create an internal, dedicated team to answering new patient phone calls with a specifically crafted script so that we were able to get more return out of our marketing dollars. Removing these operational barriers allowed us to utilize marketing dollars we were already paying for to gain more successful conversions from the new patient inquiry into patient appointments.

We have also made marketing changes in response to operational data in our practice. An example of this was when we found our marketing for patients requesting hygiene services exceeded our available rooms and staffing. At the same time, the doctor wasn't seeing ample new patients to fuel their restorative workload. This led to shifting the new patient flow to the doctor side first for the exam and x-rays and fitting the patient in same day or on another day for their cleaning. It was through viewing how we were operationally limited that we saw the opportunity to market uniquely and pivot how we framed a popular type of new patient appointment."

> Takeaways:
> - It is critical to view each location of a multi-location practice as part of the overall brand but also individually to ensure they are implementing a marketing strategy based upon that practice's needs.
> - Focus on generating marketing leads that best fit each location. While one may need hygiene patients another may need emergency or surgery patients to fill the doctor's schedule.

CHAPTER 9

What Makes a Great Practice?

I'm often asked what the best practices I work with have in common. Every great practice has an approach that works for them and their area, but there are common traits between the KPI's they monitor, the operational systems they use, and marketing strategy they rely on. The list below contains some of the common traits among the practices in this book as well as the best of best I work with.

KPI's

- The best practices track phone call data, including inbound, outbound and call answer rate. They look at when they miss the most calls and move people around to make sure they can maximize the people answering the phone. They match human resources with when the calls are coming in. This is sometimes switching people's hours around, and sometimes it's looking at specific days of the week. They also set an answer rate goal. High performing practices answer 85% or more of their calls, but the best ones are above 92%.
- They also monitor web traffic, including the number of phone and online schedule conversions from their website. These high performers know how many online scheduling appointments occur each month and know when a drop-off occurs to see potential problems.
- The best practices know the general correlation between marketing and operations. They always ask, "Can you validate the marketing numbers?" High performers do this

by comparing marketing conversions to actual new patients.
- They monitor local market share is always a big goal of the best practices. They want to maximize site visits, new patients, and production- but the visibility of the website and overall market share is the first indicator of a good practice.
- Forward Production is also a major trendline that these practices watch for. They know how well they are treatment planning and how much of that treatment planning is getting scheduled on the books for the future. If they see the treatment planning fall off, they will investigate whether the patients aren't looking for the best treatment, or whether the doctors/hygienists aren't trained enough to present best options. They know the estimated monthly revenues because they can see how much is getting scheduled over the next 2 to 4 weeks.

Operational Systems

- Top performers ensure the schedule is optimized to maximize new patient appointments. If they aren't hitting their goals, they will change the schedule around to make sure they can hit their goals, and that their goals are attainable. Sometimes block scheduling does not work, but then top performers will train their team more to ensure no one is violating new patient blocks.
- They utilize block scheduling. Block scheduling will allow patients to schedule at important intervals, and sometimes is used to just maximize the doctors' energy throughout the day.
- They always stay fully staffed. They will focus on hiring at the right times to always keep staffing at a good level- sometimes over-paying or paying above-market rates to make sure that they can keep patient flow at desired levels.
- Top performers will work to optimize the schedule for emergency patients when the hygiene schedule is full.

They know that emergency patients are just as valuable, and sometimes more valuable, than hygiene patients.
- They have a cancellation policy in place that prevents as many no shows as possible. They know cancellations also happen frequently, and they utilize an ASAP appointment list to refill patient appointments quickly.
- They have a phone script and monitor the number of new patients versus phone calls. They listen and evaluate how well staff is converting new patient calls.

Marketing Strategy

- They create and update their brand to reflect the practice. They will update their brand if they purchase an older practice, and they will make sure to match the interior decor and stylings to their brand to make everything uniform.
- They will ensure the brand represents the type of dentistry they do. Matching the name, brand, iconography, and type of dentistry is super important.
- They understand that the brand is key in increasing market share. The best practices have the highest percent of web traffic from branded searches as well as typically having the highest overall market share in their geography.
- The best practices understand that branding isn't just for the patients. Practices with a strong brand also have an advantage in hiring. People want to work for a practice that they connect with.
- The best practices never sign long term contracts that tie them into financial obligations. They will ensure the marketing is versatile and nimble to allow for changes when needed.
- They create an online foundation and determine how much effort and resources they need for digital marketing. All practices need an online presence but not all need to spend the same.

When a practice matches KPIs with operations and a solid marketing strategy, it creates a flywheel of success that is hard to stop. I've seen it many times, and thus, while writing it was a challenge to select a handful of dental practices to highlight. When practices get this trifecta correct, they tend to reach their goals of new patient acquisition, increasing their active patient base, production per patient and overall, an increase in their revenue.

I hope that in reading this book, you gained perspective on how important marketing and operations are connected to each other and how you should use your operation numbers to validate your marketing. Anyone can spend money on marketing but without a strategy that is built around your practice and for your market, you may be spending money with little to no ROI. I hope this book showcases the importance of connection between operations and marketing and allows you to pave the way for owning an exceptional dental practice with a momentum that is unstoppable!

Made in the USA
Monee, IL
05 June 2023